KEGEL EXERCISES FOR MEN

STEP BY STEP GUIDE ON KEGEL EXERCISES FOR MEN TO LAST LONGER IN BED, TREAT ERECTILE DYSFUNCTION AND URINARY INCONTINENCE FOR OPTIMUM PROSTRATE HEALTH

By

Michael Irwin

Copyright @2018

CONTENTS

Introduction 1

Chapter 1 5

Benefits of Kegel Exercises 5

   1. For Urinary Incontinence 5

   2. For Anal Incontinence 6

   3. For Overactive Bladder 7

   4. For Healthy Prostate 9

   5. For Sexual Performance Anxiety . 9

Chapter 2 13

What to Do Before You Start Your Kegel Exercises 13

   How to Start Performing Your Kegel Exercises 16

Chapter 3 21

How To Get The Best Results And A Cool Kegel Device 21

A Cool Kegel Device 27

Chapter 4 29

What You Should Know About Reverse Kegels 29

Conclusion 31

Introduction

Here's a quick quiz:

Question 1: True or false, Kegel exercises are beneficial

Question 2: True or false, you know what to do before you start your Kegel exercises

Question 3: True or false, you know how to start performing your Kegel exercises properly

Question 4: True or false, you know how to get the best results from your Kegels

If you answered "true" to at least two of these questions, pat yourself on the back – you know quite a bit about Kegels.

If you got anyone wrong, there's still more you need to learn.

It's not your fault if you don't know the benefits of Kegels, or perhaps you don't even know how to perform it properly. That's because there's a lot of contradictory information floating around about Kegels.

Good news is, you're here to learn all you need to know about Kegel exercises for men in this book.

You will discover:

- Benefits of Kegel exercises
- What to do before you start your Kegel exercises
- How to get the best results and a cool Kegel device
- What you should know about reverse Kegels

So roll up your sleeves, put on your thinking cap, and let's delve into the world of Kegels...

Chapter 1

Benefits of Kegel Exercises

Here are the benefits of Kegel exercises for six different health issues:

1. For Urinary Incontinence

When the muscles connecting your bladder and urinary tract are weak, you will experience urinary incontinence - passing out of urine uncontrollably. This is usually noticeable after working out, coughing, laughing or even standing from a seating position.

In some cases, you may experience dribbling - urine leakage after urination. But a strong pelvic floor muscle can prevent urinary incontinence, and with Kegel exercises, you can build strong pelvic floor muscles.

2. For Anal Incontinence

You can improve your ability to manage your anal incontinence by improving the tone and strength of your anal sphincter and the muscles that surround it (including your pelvic floor muscles) through Kegel exercises. Also, if you usually have anal sex, Kegel exercises can be beneficial in strengthening your sphincter muscles to improve its tone.

3. For Overactive Bladder

If you always have the urge or the need to use the restroom constantly, then, it is highly likely that you have an over-active bladder. It is a conditioned response that can be triggered when you hear running water or enter a bathroom.

When that conditioned response is triggered, there is a contraction of the muscles surrounding your bladder which triggers a squeezing effect and creates the urge in you to urinate. Kegel exercises that can help you to prevent these involuntary contractions since the stronger your pelvic muscles, the greater the control you will have over your muscles.

4. For Healthy Prostate

Since Kegel exercises also improve blood circulation within the body, these exercises can help you to maintain a strong prostate health and manage prostate enlargement symptoms.

5. For Sexual Performance Anxiety

Sexual performance anxiety is a sexual distress due to the combination of biological, psychological and social factors.

When you're stressed and anxious, your body generates adrenaline and cortisol both of which inhibits penile circulation. The psychological factor entails nervousness and previous negative sexual experience. Socially, you are worried about being ashamed or embarrassed by your partner due to your bad sexual performance. Other factors can be work, relationship, and family issues.

However, it is a proven fact that any exercise that improves sexual health usually inspire self-confidence. For example, if you are trying to lose weight through intermittent fasting, the first day of fast won't make you lose weight. Rather, it will create a positive mindset in you and give you a renewed self-belief.

This same principle applies to the use of Kegels to remedy performance anxiety. Although, bear in mind that relying on Kegels alone to solve your deep-seated anxieties won't be effective.

Chapter 2

What to Do Before You Start Your Kegel Exercises

You need to find your pelvic muscles before you can start performing your Kegels. Stopping the flow of your urine midway is one of the most common ways to find your pelvic muscles. However, if you have any medical issues, consult your doctor before starting to perform your Kegels.

But don't include stopping your urine midway as part of your Kegel routine because this might weaken your muscle and damage your bladder and kidneys.

Also, you shouldn't start your Kegels with a full bladder. If you do, you will experience pain during your Kegels.

For the best results, your Kegel exercises should focus on tightening your pelvic floor muscles. Also, rather than hold your breath, exhale and inhale while performing each Kegels set. This will improve the effectiveness of your movements and your concentration. If you experience any pain after completing a set of Kegel exercises, it is likely that you're doing your Kegel exercises the wrong way.

Lastly, perform your Kegels while seated or lying back down. Then, relax your tummy and buttock muscles. If you are lying down, your back should be flat, your arms by your sides, your knees up and your head down to prevent neck strain.

How to Start Performing Your Kegel Exercises

- Start by squeezing your pelvic muscles for three seconds. If you squeeze those muscles longer than three seconds, you might strain them and cause more harm than any good.
- Release your pelvic muscles for 5 seconds, then, repeat step one. You can count from one to five before repeating step one. This break will prevent any strain to the pelvic muscles.

- Repeat steps one and two 15 times. This is one Kegel set - squeeze muscles for three seconds, release for five seconds and repeat for fifteen times.

When you are just starting, you should only perform a maximum of three Kegel sets per day. But each week, continue to increase your squeeze and relax time till you reach a squeeze time of ten seconds and a relax time of fifteen seconds. But do not perform more than four Kegel sets per day.

After reaching a squeeze time of ten seconds, maintain it for up to three weeks before making any changes. Once you've mastered the squeeze and hold technique, you can start to perform the pull-in technique. This technique is done by lying back down with your buttocks tense, but your legs pulled up and in. Maintain that position for five seconds before relaxing your body. Repeat this ten times successively to complete the whole reps in fifty seconds.

Alternately, after you've mastered the squeeze and hold technique, you can start performing fast Kegels rather than increasing your squeeze and relax periods. The only difference between the fast Kegels and the squeeze and hold Kegel is the relaxation period.

Here's a simple and fast Kegel exercise you can perform:

- Squeeze those muscles for five seconds.

- Release them for 2 seconds, count one to two, then, repeat.
- Repeat steps one and two 10 times to make one Kegel set

Chapter 3

How To Get The Best Results And A Cool Kegel Device

Once you start performing your Kegel sets four times per day, do not skip any day. Since each Kegel session doesn't take a long time, you should find a way to fit your Kegels into your daily activities. You can schedule your Kegels for morning, afternoon, evening and night to make it easy for you when you're just getting started.

Since Kegels are simple and easy to perform, you can perform them without the knowledge of anyone. You can perform them while relaxing on your couch after a day's work, during lunch with your colleagues and friends, or in your office while seated at your desk. When you're just getting started, the number one hindrance to performing your Kegels properly would be your inability to locate your pelvic floor muscles.

But once it's easy for you to locate those muscles, it would be easy for you to perform your Kegels at any time of the day. If you perform your Kegels regularly and properly, it should take about three months before you start getting any results. Don't stop performing Kegels because you failed to get results within a few weeks. Yes, some people might start getting results within a few weeks (some as early as four weeks), but not everyone is going to get results within a few weeks.

If after six months of performing Kegels and there are no signs of improvement, your best option is to consult your doctor. It is either you are performing the exercise the wrong way (you are targeting wrong muscles), or your body is not suited for the exercise.

Here's what you can expect from your doctor: your doctor can help you to identify your pelvic floor muscles using electrical stimulation. The electrical simulation technique involves passing a minute electrical current through your pelvic floor muscles. Those muscles automatically contract when the current passes through it. Over time, you should be able to start contracting those muscles by yourself.

Once your doctor has helped you to identify those muscles, you should continue to perform your Kegels until you start getting the results you desire. If you stop after a few weeks, your sexual health might deteriorate.

While you may be tempted to think that increasing the pace of your Kegel routines when you're just starting will strengthen your muscles faster, this is not true at all. The fact is, excessive Kegel reps and sets can weaken your pelvic muscles. Hence, worsening your sexual health rather than improve it.

If you follow the recommendations (performing the exercises as described, breathing normally during the exercise, relaxing other muscles of your body during the exercise and performing the exercise on an empty bladder), performing Kegels has no side effect. If you perform Kegels when your bladder is full or even partially full, you might have urinary tract infections.

If you find it impossible to breathe during your Kegels, I suggest you breathe in as you squeeze the muscles, and breathe out as you release the contraction.

A Cool Kegel Device

The Kgoal Boost is a popular device that can improve the performance of your pelvic floor exercises, prevent bladder leaks and improve your sexual strength. It is a pulsating button which you have to sit upon either in your car, office, church pew or on your couch. Since it can connect with your smartphone app, it guides you on various activities (which doesn't exceed five minutes) to exercise your pelvic muscles.

Chapter 4

What You Should Know About Reverse Kegels

Just like the name, reverse Kegels are the opposite of the standard Kegels. While in a standard Kegel, you have to contract and release your pelvic floor muscles, in a reverse Kegel, you have to release and relax your pelvic floor muscles.

Reverse Kegels offers the same benefits as standard Kegels. Also, you need to exercise the same precautions as standard Kegels, while you can expect results between four weeks and six months.

Conclusion

With the enormous health benefits of Kegel exercises, nothing stops you from incorporating Kegel exercises into your daily routine. Combining Kegel exercises with sitting properly, standing up straight and walking properly can strengthen your pelvic floor muscles quicker.

The whole point of this book was to make you realize the benefits of Kegels and how to perform them properly. Indeed, you started out thinking there may not be any benefits of doing Kegel exercises; I hope by now that you've come to realize Kegels are beneficial and you can perform them easily.

I don't necessarily expect you to start combining reverse and standard Kegels. Rather, it would be helpful if you start with the Kegel sets as described in Chapter 2.

However, you can build strong pelvic floor muscles through a combination of the reverse and standard Kegels.

Let me leave you with this quote:

"Take time to deliberate; but when the time for action arrives, stop thinking and go in." - Andrew Jackson

So, go all in right now.

www.ingramcontent.com/pod-product-compliance
Lightning Source LLC
Chambersburg PA
CBHW030119230526
45469CB00005B/1715